The Keto Thanksgiving Cookbook

HOW TO HAVE A KETO THANKSGIVING WITH TWENTY-TWO EASY RECIPES

By Tara G. Wright

Follow Tara's Keto Kitchen on social
- ☑ YouTube
- ☑ Instagram
- ☑ Facebook
- ☑ Pinterest

Introduction

"When I first started the Keto Diet, I knew I had to figure out how to make keto alternatives to our favorite foods. So many of the staple ingredients are taboo and there wasn't a lot of information on the science of keto ingredients. I had a real challenge on my hands."

~Health Coach Tara

Learning to cook keto is counterintuitive but certainly not impossible. I decided to start Tara's Keto Kitchen after trying about a dozen keto recipes that turned out so badly they went right in the garbage.

Keto ingredients were expensive and I knew that if I put my mind to it and was willing to experiment, I could figure out how to cook with these new ingredients. After all, I've been baking and cooking since I was a wee bairn. I first learned in my great grandmother's kitchen. Later on, I took all the cooking classes my high school offered and started creating my own recipes.

When I converted to a keto lifestyle, my greatest challenge was figuring out how to use grain-free flours and keto ingredients to get baked goods to turn out perfectly every time.

As the holidays approached, I started experimenting with different Thanksgiving dishes as early as September. The pie crust in this e-book took me two years to get just right. You'll want to make sure you use pie crust shields when you bake the crust so the edges don't come out dark brown.

To learn more about sugar substitutes, visit our website at wholebodyliving.com. Then search for 'sugar substitute' and you will find the guide I keep updated with the most current information. My hope for you this holiday season is that you can enjoy delicious food and be surrounded by those who love you.

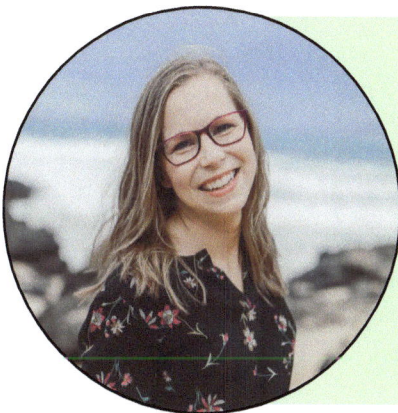

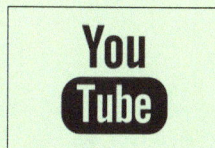

You
Tube

Health Coach Tara
YouTube.com/TarasKetoKitchen
wholebodyliving.com

Discover tools to help make keto easier including planners, tear-off pads, and more. Shop our store at sustainableketo.com.

How To Have A Low-Carb Thanksgiving

This cookbook is our complete Thanksgiving dinner menu and we hope you enjoy it as much as we do. Here's some tips for having a low-carb Thanksgiving without shocking your body out of ketosis.

TIP #1: THE LONGER YOU'VE BEEN IN KETOSIS, THE MORE CARBS YOU CAN EAT

Once your body becomes fat-adapted, you gain the added flexibility of being able to allow more carbs into your diet while remaining in ketosis. This comes in especially handy during the holidays.

The amount of carbs you can allow yourself is going to vary greatly from person to person.

Aim for about 20% carbs, 60-70% fat and 10-20% protein. I've personally been able to stay in ketosis after I became fat adapted eating as high as 30% carbohydrates.

TIP #2: USE INTERMITTENT FASTING AS YOUR SUPERPOWER

If you've never fasted before, start today. I have a video on YouTube (search Tara's Keto Kitchen Intermittent Fasting on YouTube) about how to get started.

There's a few ways you can harness the power of fasting for Thanksgiving:

Option 1: Fast on Thanksgiving Day until dinner and make this your only meal.

Option 2: Begin fasting immediately after your Thanksgiving Dinner and fast for 16-24 hours. Allow water only after dinner. You can have coffee with 1 Tablespoon heavy cream before breaking your fast in the morning.

Repeat until your tests show you're back in ketosis.

TIP #3: TRAVELING FOR THANKSGIVING? PLAN AHEAD

Whether you're going to be in the car or on a plane, planning ahead makes staying low-carb much easier.

Pack a small cooler in your carry-on with some of your favorite keto snacks. Low-carb nuts, slices of cheese, pork rinds, homemade keto crackers or chips, string cheese, and sugar-free meat sticks are a few ideas to get you started.

If you're terrible at planning - decide you'll figure it out and follow through on that commitment. Explore our line of keto planners, meal planning worksheets, and more at sustainableketo.com.

Large airports and gas stations always have a low-carb option to choose from. Keep in mind that some things will be closed if you're traveling ON Thanksgiving. If you really want to stay low-carb, then plan ahead.

TIP #4 CONSIDER A "BREAK" FOR A DAY

If you're attending a big function where you'll have zero control over food, just choose the healthiest options possible and allow yourself a ONE DAY break.

This doesn't mean you should stuff yourself so full you can't move. This doesn't mean you're going to stuff yourself from now until January 1st. This does means you'll take a break for a specific time period.

This is a strategy called carb cycling and it can be very good for your body when you do it right. Get in some extra activity and enjoy the family & friends you're surrounded with. Happy Thanksgiving!

CONTENTS

Keto Hot Cocoa Mix

I created this recipe so we would have a special treat while getting our Christmas tree the day after Thanksgiving. There's just something about hot cocoa that brings back the best holiday memories. Choose a MCT powder with acacia fiber or gum acacia. If the label doesn't say what kind of fiber is used in the MCT powder, move on to a different brand.

1 cup unsweetened cocoa powder
½ cup MCT powder
½ cup sugar substitute
1 Tablespoon black cocoa powder (optional)
½ teaspoon fine sea salt

Mix all ingredients together until completely combined and there are no clumps.

Store in an airtight container until ready to use.

To make keto hot cocoa, blend 2 Tablespoons hot cocoa mix with 6 ounces warmed milk alternative or hot water. Top with real whipped cream.

30 CAL | 11.7 G CARB | 4.2 G FIBER | 1.3 G NET CARB | 3 G FAT | 1 G PROTEIN

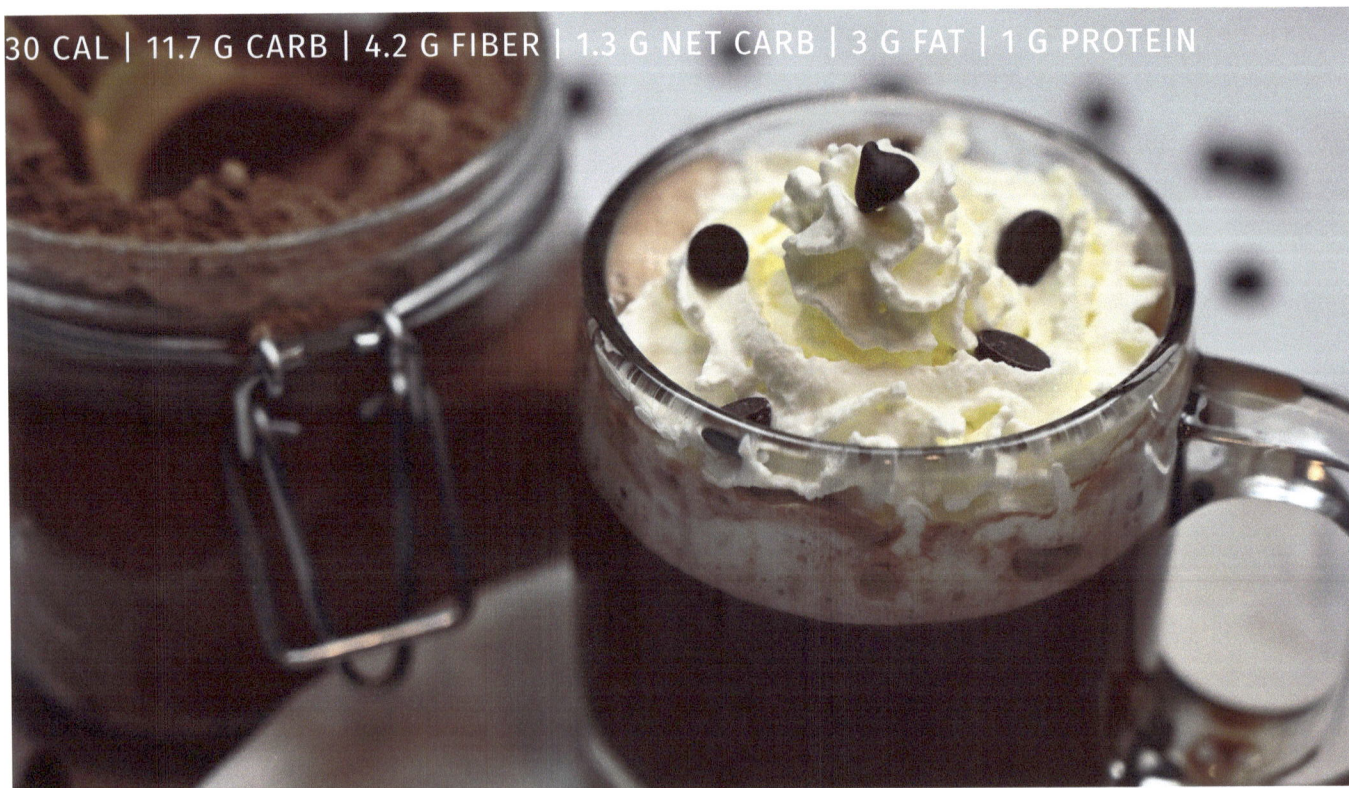

Low-Carb Sangria

Enjoy a glass of sangria with your Thanksgiving dinner with this easy to make recipe. Your friends and family won't have any idea it's low-carb. Vary the flavors of your sangria by trying different fruit teas and different dry red wine blends until you find your favorite combination.

1 bottle dry red wine
2 cups strongly brewed fruit tea
1 lime, sliced
⅔ cup sugar substitute

Cut a lemon or lime into slices.

Brew a strong fruit tea of your choosing.

In a large pitcher, mix together the tea with the sugar substitute while the tea is still warm. This allows it to dissolve faster. If the tea is already cold, it will just take a few minutes of mixing to get the sweetener to dissolve.

Drop the lime into the tea mixture and muddle for a few minutes using a wooden spoon.

Next, mix in the dry red wine. Pour slowly so you don't splatter the wine.

Chill your sangria for 2 to 12 hours and enjoy over ice.

(NO NUTRITION FACTS AS IT WILL VARY BASED ON THE WINE CHOSEN)

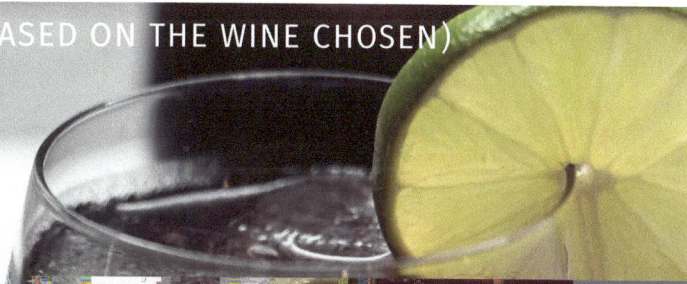

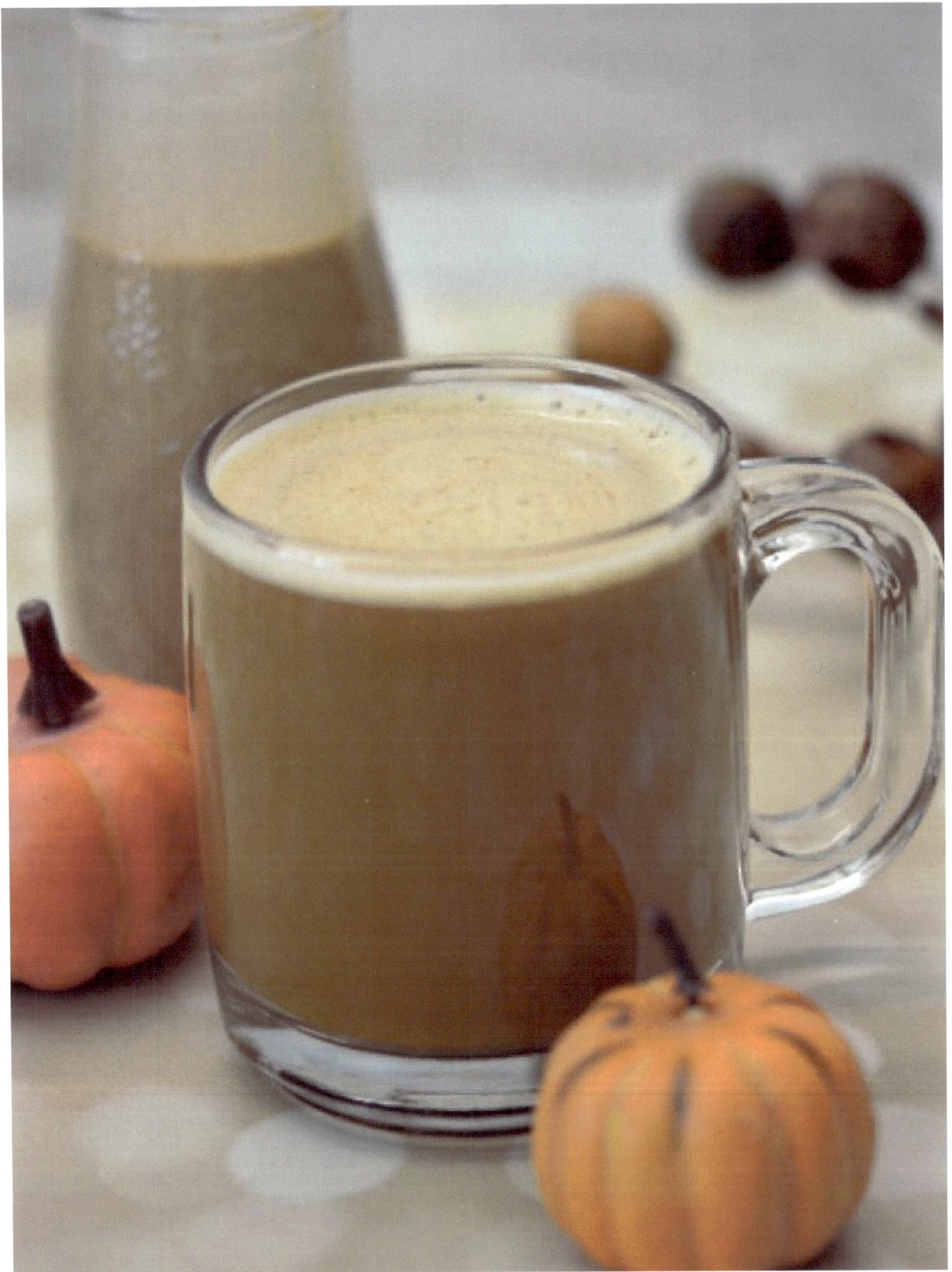

Pumpkin Spice Coffee Creamer

1 can (15 ounces) unsweetened coconut milk

1 Tablespoon pumpkin pie spice

⅓ cup granulated sugar substitute

3 Tablespoons MCT oil

1 Tablespoon pure vanilla extract

¼ cup pumpkin puree

In a small saucepan, heat a few inches of water over low heat. Place the unopened can of coconut milk in the pan with the top down. (The coconut cream hardens on top of the coconut milk in the can. Turn the heat down to low and let the coconut milk warm for about five minutes while you assemble the remaining ingredients.

In a medium sized bowl, mix remaining ingredients until combined.

Carefully remove warmed coconut milk from heat (the can may be hot) and shake vigorously to combine the coconut cream with the milk.

Mix the warmed coconut milk into the pumpkin base.

Store in a tightly sealed container in the fridge for up to one week.

43 CAL | .5 G NET CARB | 4.4 G FAT | .1 G PROTEIN

There's nothing quite like the fresh taste of pumpkin spice in your coffee on Thanksgiving morning.

To make your creamer with dairy, substitute the canned coconut milk with:

1 cup heavy whipping cream

½ cup distilled water

In the recipe above, skip the instructions for warming the milk. You can simply combine all the ingredients and mix them together.

Store in a tightly sealed container in the fridge until the sell by date on your carton of cream.

50 CAL | .5 G NET CARB | 5.4 G FAT | .3 G PROTEIN

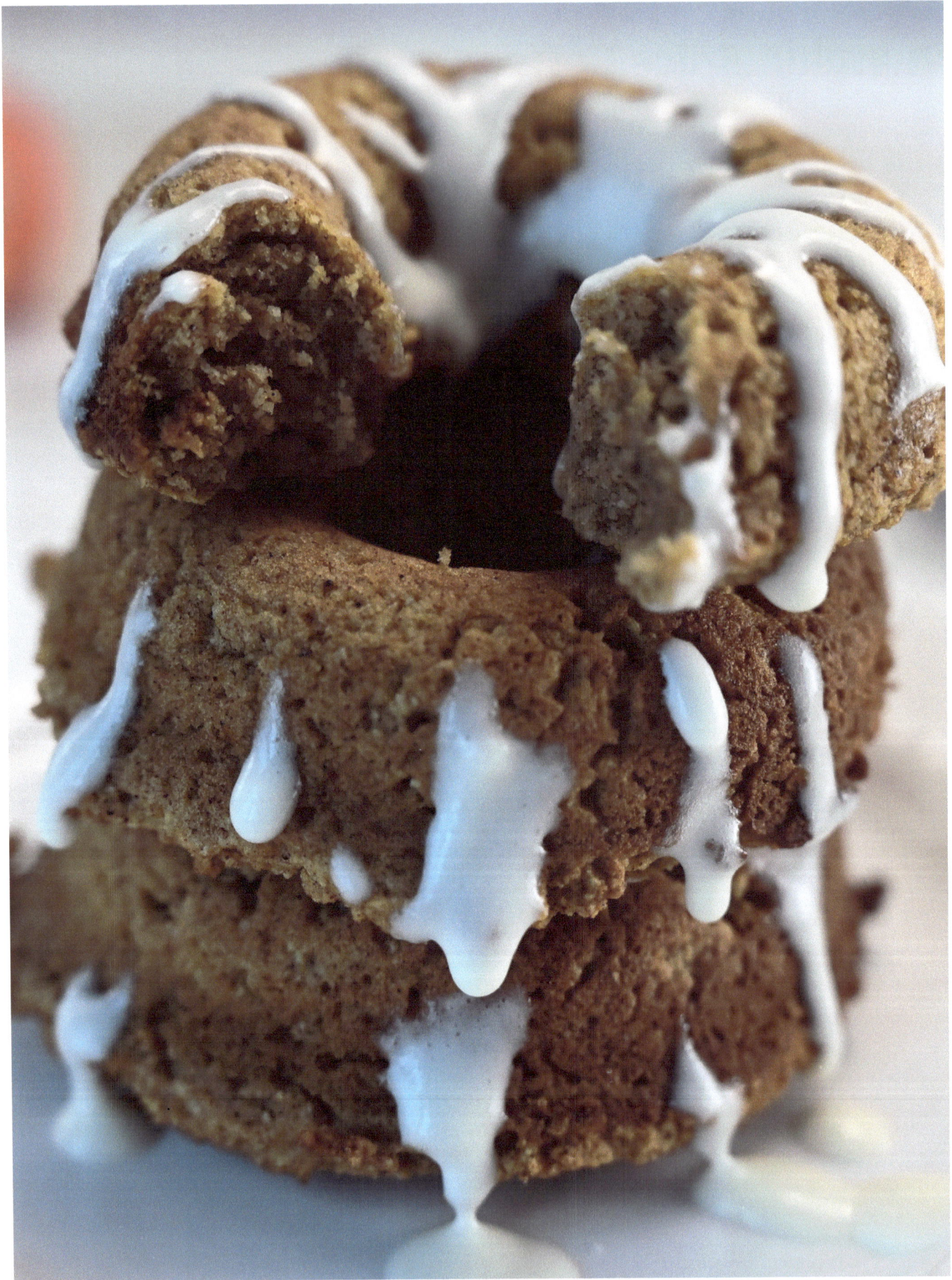

Keto Pumpkin Spice Donuts

These low-carb pumpkin spice donuts are a crowd-pleaser. You will need a donut pan to make these. To make the glaze, mix together a tablespoon of heavy cream (or coconut cream), a tablespoon of melted butter, 1/2 teaspoon vanilla, and two tablespoons of sugar substitute. Mix until the sugar substitute is dissolved and then drizzle over cooled donuts.

6 Tablespoons avocado oil

3 eggs

⅓ cup heavy cream

½ cup pumpkin puree

¾ cup sugar substitute

1 ½ teaspoon vanilla extract

1 Tablespoon pumpkin pie spice

1 ½ teaspoon cinnamon

1 cup (113 g) coconut flour

1 ½ teaspoon baking powder

¾ teaspoon xanthan gum

¾ teaspoon salt

Preheat oven to 325 °F.

Prepare donut pan by generously greasing it with coconut oil or avocado oil.

In a medium-sized mixing bowl combine the avocado oil, eggs, heavy cream, pumpkin puree, sugar substitute, vanilla extract, pumpkin pie spice, and cinnamon. Blend on low speed until completely combined and smooth.

In a small bowl, mix together coconut flour, xanthan gum, baking powder, and salt. Stir to combine.

Mix the coconut flour mixture into the pumpkin mixture until completely combined. Allow mixture to rest for 5 minutes. The batter will thicken considerably.

Then, fill the cups of ten donuts in your donut pan. The donuts will rise as they bake.

Bake at 325 °F for 20-25 minutes or until a toothpick inserted into the center comes out clean.

Remove from oven and allow to cool for 5-10 minutes before removing from the pan.

182 CAL | 14.4 G FAT | 21.5 G CARB | 12.5 G SUGAR ALCOHOL
4.2 G NET CARB | 4.8 G FIBER | 3.9 G PROTEIN

Keto Deviled Eggs

Thanksgiving wouldn't be complete without deviled eggs on the table. Our favorite way to hard-boil large eggs is to add them to boiling water and then boil for 14 minutes. Remove the eggs from the pan and immediately place in an ice bath so they cool rapidly. Store in a carton until ready to make deviled eggs.

12 large hard-boiled eggs

¾ cup mayonnaise

⅛ cup yellow mustard

¼ teaspoon salt

¼ teaspoon white pepper or lemon pepper

Paprika to garnish

Start with cooled, peeled hard-boiled eggs.

Cut each egg in half longwise and remove the yolk from the egg white. Place yolks in a small bowl that will be good for mashing.

Mash the egg yolks in your bowl with a fork until you have very small pieces of mashed yolk.

Stir in mayonnaise, mustard, salt, and pepper.

Mix until completely combined.

Fill each egg white shell with the egg mixture.

Eat immediately or store covered in the fridge for 1-2 days.

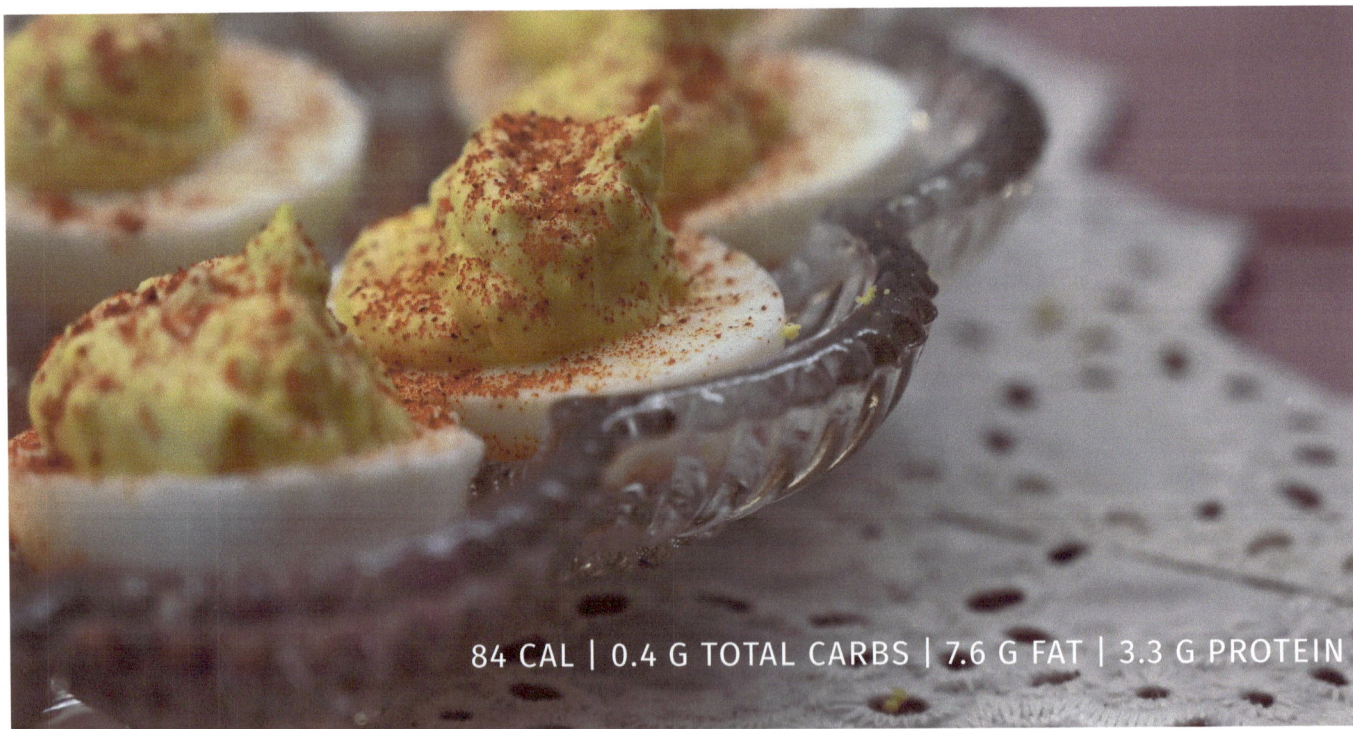

84 CAL | 0.4 G TOTAL CARBS | 7.6 G FAT | 3.3 G PROTEIN

Keto Mashed "Potatoes"

Rich, silky, and luxurious - you won't even notice that you're eating cauliflower instead of mashed potatoes. If you're feeding a crowd, you'll want to double this recipe. If there are any leftovers, we like to use them as a base to make leftover Thanksgiving "bowls" to eat the next day. Start by putting these in the bottom of a bowl, and then add your favorite leftovers on top. Heat and enjoy.

Two, 16 ounces packages riced cauliflower
4 ounces cream cheese
1 teaspoon salt

Cook riced cauliflower according to package directions.

Puree all ingredients together in a food processor until smooth.

Serve with toppings of your choice. Shown with herbed butter.

84 CAL | 0.4 G TOTAL CARBS | 7.6 G FAT | 3.3 G PROTEIN

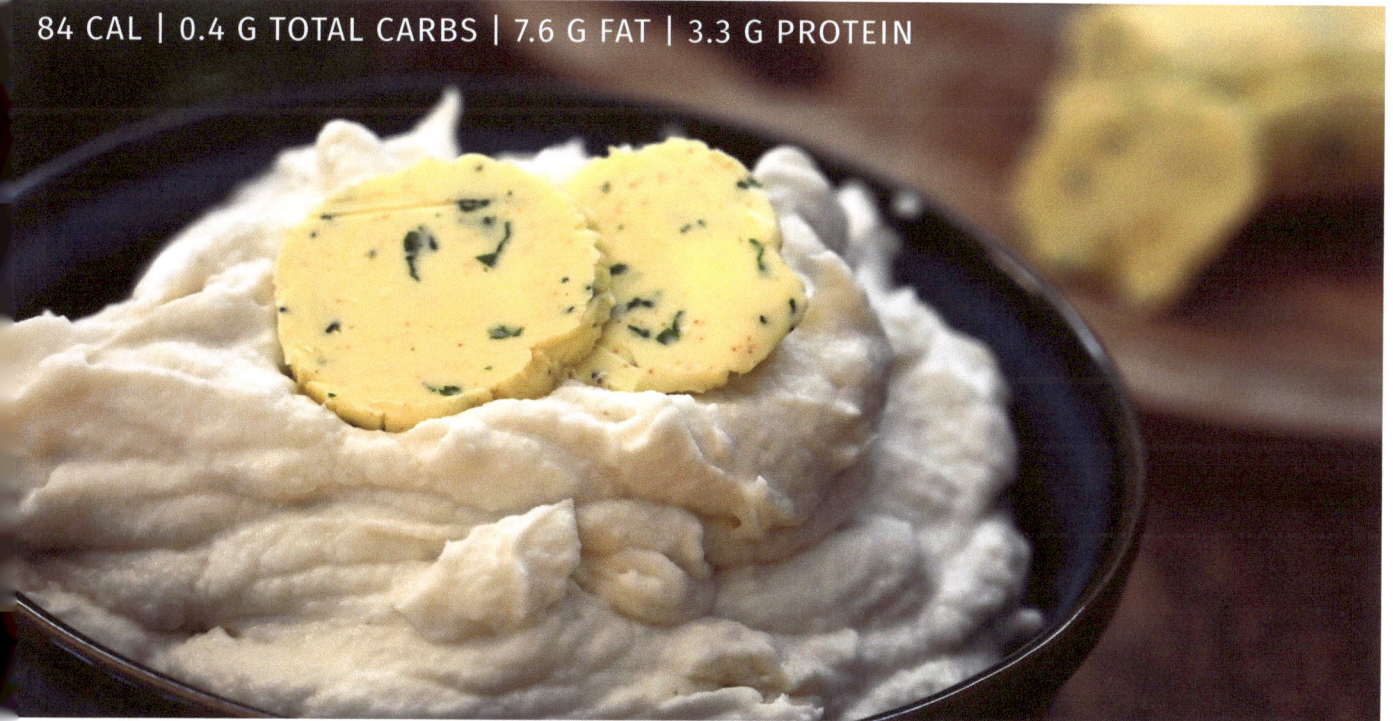

Herbed Butter

This simple herbed butter will dress up your Thanksgiving table. Use any fresh herbs you enjoy. Our favorite combination is parsley and dill.

½ cup butter (1 stick)
1 Tablespoon fresh minced parsley
½ Tablespoon fresh minced dill
⅛ teaspoon garlic powder
¼ teaspoon salt

Soften your butter and mix in the herbs and salt. Mix together until well combined.

Place butter mixture in saran wrap. Wrap and mold butter into a log. You can also mold the butter using butter or candy molds if you wish.

Place herbed butter in the refrigerator to harden for at least an hour.

Unwrap, slice & serve.

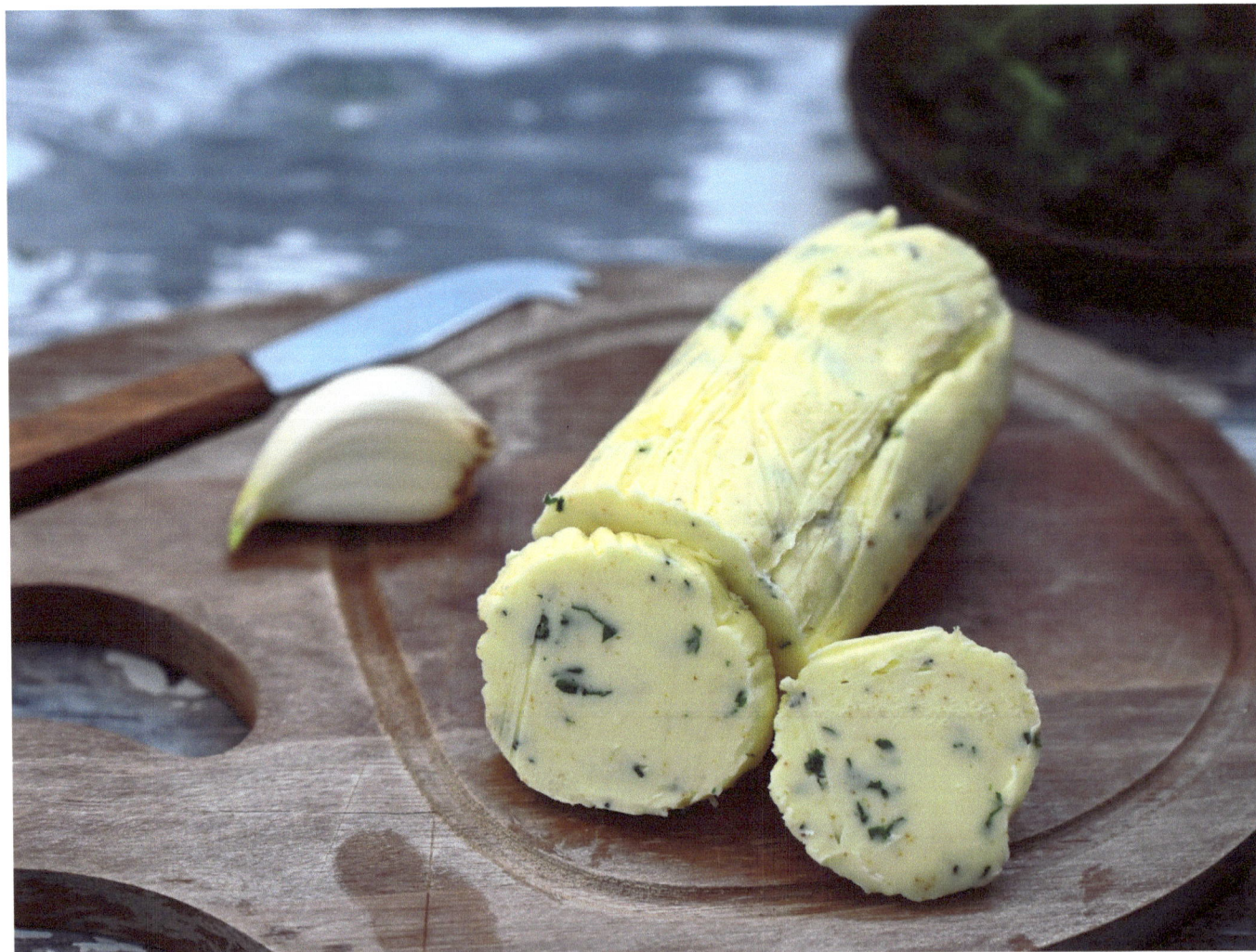

Keto Pull-Apart Rolls

These rolls are a family tradition on our holiday table. As kids, my sisters and I loved rolling the dough balls and putting them into a cupcake pan. There's nothing like pulling them apart at dinner time. This keto version is our new family favorite. You can make them the day ahead or make them weeks in advance and store them in your freezer.

2 cups (226 g) whole milk mozzarella, shredded

2 ounces cream cheese

2 eggs, large

1 Tablespoon gelatin

1 ¼ cup (140 g) almond flour

1 Tablespoon coconut flour

2 teaspoons baking powder

In a medium-sized microwave-safe bowl, microwave mozzarella and cream cheese for one minute. Remove from the microwave and stir to combine. If the mozzarella isn't quite melted, return to the microwave for twenty seconds and stir. Do not overheat the mixture. Set this cheese mixture aside to cool.

In a large mixing bowl, crack eggs into the bottom of the bowl and whisk until combined. Then, while still whisking, sprinkle in the gelatin and whisk vigorously until light and foamy. You can also use your electric blender for this step. Stop and scrape down the sides of the bowl as needed.

Using your blender, or upper body strength, mix in the melted cheese until completely combined.

Then, blend in the almond flour, coconut flour, and baking powder.

Place the dough in the refrigerator for 20-30 minutes.

In the meantime, preheat the oven to 375 °F. Then, prepare cupcake pans by greasing the inside of each cup with coconut oil.

Once the dough has chilled, divide into 12 portions. Take each of these portions and divide them into thirds. Using your hands, roll each third into a ball. Place three balls into each cup of your cupcake pan.

Bake in a preheated oven for 10-12 minutes until golden on top and bottom and cooked through.

Remove from the oven and allow to cool for at least 5 minutes before enjoying.

Recipe Tips: If you can't find whole milk mozzarella, use 1 cup part-skim mozzarella and 1 cup white cheddar cheese. (You can also use orange cheddar but the rolls will be yellow in color). The gelatin can be replaced with 1 teaspoon xanthan gum with similar results.

161 CALORIES | 3.7 G CARB | 1.5 G FIBER

2.1 G NET CARB | 13.1 G FAT | 8.4 G PROTEIN

Keto Dinner Rolls

Coconut flour makes light and fluffy rolls with just a hint of coconut flavor. Consider adding a half teaspoon of garlic powder if you are sensitive to the slight coconut flavor of the flour.

½ cup (56 g) coconut flour
1 teaspoon baking powder
½ teaspoon xanthan gum
½ teaspoon salt
1 Tablespoon avocado oil
4 large eggs
1 Tablespoon gelatin
½ cup warm water

Preheat your oven to 350 °F in a standard oven.

In a medium sized mixing bowl, combine the coconut flour, baking powder, xanthan gum, and salt.

In a small glass mixing bowl, whisk eggs together and sprinkle in gelatin while still stirring. Stir in the gelatin until no clumps remain and egg mixture has thickened, about one minute.

Pour the warm water into the coconut flour mixture and stir just until the coconut flour soaks up the water. Pour in the egg mixture and mix with a spatula to incorporate all the ingredients thoroughly, about one minute. Make sure there are no clumps.

Allow the mixture to sit for 5 minutes while you prepare a baking sheet by lightly greasing it or covering with parchment paper.

Divide rolls into six equal parts and roll into a ball. Place on the baking sheet. Cut an X into the top of the roll if desired.

Bake for 25-30 minutes until golden brown and set up in the middle. Enjoy hot and fresh out of the oven or make the day ahead and warm up in the oven before your meal.

117 CALORIES | 6.1 G CARB | 3.5 G FIBER | 2.6 G NET CARB | 7.1 G FAT | 6.5 G PROTEIN

Creamy Keto Green Bean Casserole

This creamy green bean casserole is so good, you won't miss the real thing. We've used crush pork rinds instead of onions on top to mimic the crunchy texture of the original casserole. Sour cream, coconut aminos, and seasonings take the place of cream of mushroom soup. You might want to double this recipe.

2 cans (14 ½ ounces each) green beans
½ teaspoon onion powder
¼ teaspoon salt
½ teaspoon ground black pepper
1 Tablespoon coconut aminos
  or liquid aminos
1 cup sour cream
4 ounces shredded sharp cheddar cheese
½ cup crushed pork rinds

Preheat oven to 350 °F.

Prepare a 9x9 casserole dish by greasing the bottom and sides.

Combine sour cream, onion powder, salt, black pepper, and coconut aminos in a medium size bowl. Stir until combined.

Mix in the green beans and shredded cheese.

Place pork rinds in a sturdy plastic bag and crush with a rolling pin.

Sprinkle crushed pork rinds on top of the casserole.

Bake at 350 °F for 40 minutes or until bubbling in the center.

201 CAL | 5.5 G NET CARB | 14.3 G FAT | 7.9 G PROTEIN

Turkey Gravy

This gravy goes great over the top of your dark meat turkey & mashed cauliflower potatoes.

1 cup turkey drippings ¼ teaspoon xanthan gum	Making grain-free gravy is easy if you have some xanthan gum on hand. You can use either turkey drippings, broth, or a mixture of the two. You'll need 1/4 teaspoon xanthan gum per cup of liquid. In a saucepan over medium heat, combine turkey drippings and xanthan gum, whisking vigorously. I like to use my immersion blender when I add the xanthan gum so I don't get any clumping. You can also pour the mixture into a blender before heating and blend the two together, then put it in the pan to simmer. Bring to a simmer and cook for about 5 minutes until thickened. Serve while warm or make the day ahead and re-heat when needed.

No Sugar Added Cranberry Sauce

My husband's favorite part of Thanksgiving is the cranberry sauce. Fortunately, cranberries are a low-sugar keto friendly berry. Here, we use two different sugar substitutes to provide the best flavor possible. Using the orange rind is optional, but I always include it.

16 ounces whole cranberries

30 drops liquid stevia

1 Tablespoon granulated sugar substitute

¼ teaspoon almond extract

½ cup water

2 pieces orange rind

In a medium-sized saucepan, over low heat, dissolve granulated sugar substitute in water.

Add the cranberries and orange rind and slowly bring to a boil over medium-high heat. The cranberries will begin to pop as they heat.

Once cranberries begin to "pop", reduce heat to medium and simmer for 20-25 minutes until the sauce has thickened. Stir every few minutes.

Now it's time to add the finishing touches. Stir in almond extract and liquid stevia drops. I like to start with 15 drops of stevia and then taste test it, adding more until I'm pleased with the finished results.

Let your cranberry sauce cool and store in a tightly sealed container for up to one week.

8 CAL | 2 G NET CARB | 0 G FAT | 0 G PROTEIN

Sugar Free Maple Bourbon Glaze

This bourbon glaze will work with any sugar substitute. If you prefer to make the glaze without the bourbon just substitute water for the bourbon and you're good to go.

¼ cup water

½ cup BochaSweet

1 Tablespoon butter

¼ cup granulated sugar substitute

1 Tablespoon dijon mustard

¼ cup bourbon

¼ teaspoon allspice

½ teaspoon maple extract

⅛ teaspoon xanthan gum

In a small saucepan over low heat, stir together water and BochaSweet until granules are completely dissolved.

Remove pan from heat and whisk in the remaining ingredients.

Be careful adding the xanthan gum because it tends to clump. You may need to use a blender or a immersion blender to completely mix in the xanthan gum. It can be tricky.

This glaze can be used on ham, salmon, chicken, pork, and fish.

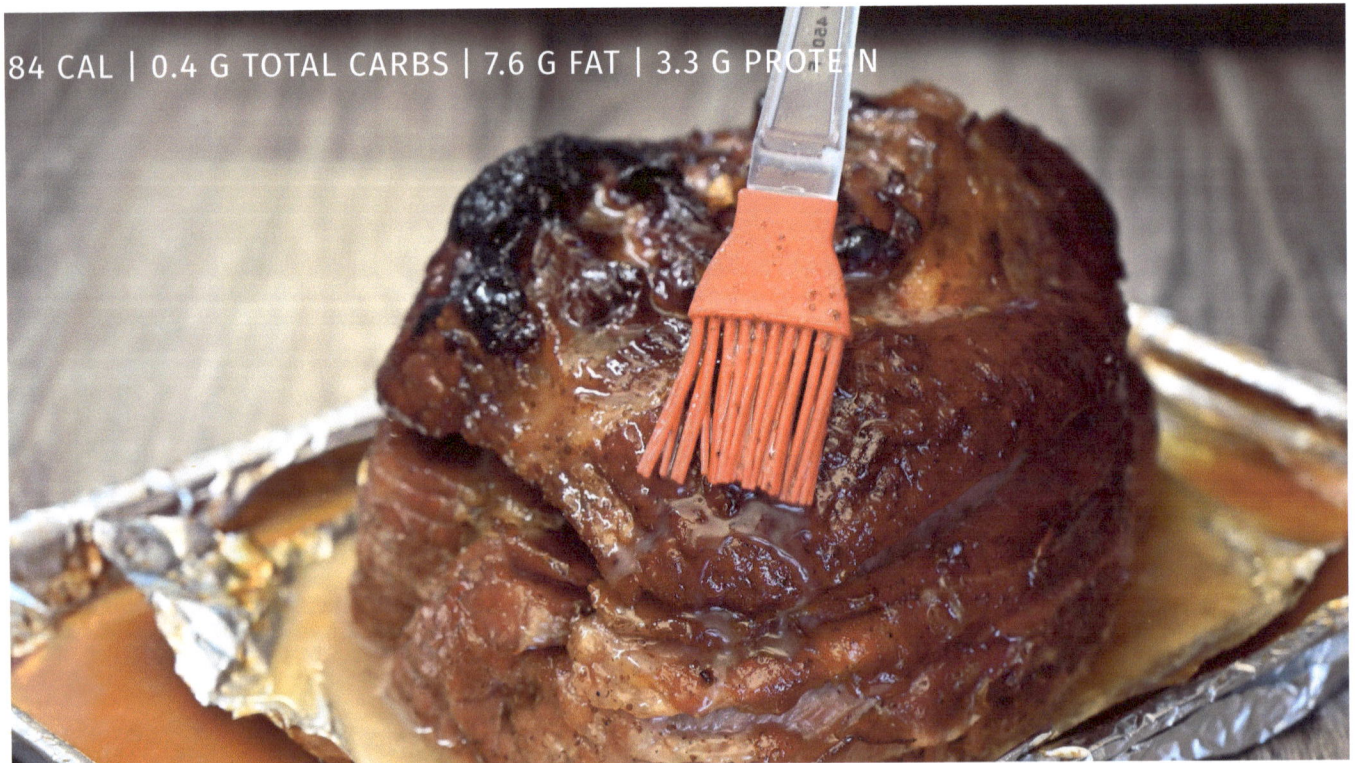

84 CAL | 0.4 G TOTAL CARBS | 7.6 G FAT | 3.3 G PROTEIN

Sugar Free Maple Bourbon Glazed Ham

You can still have a traditional glazed ham at your Thanksgiving table. Here, I'll show you how to use the maple bourbon glaze to create a delicious Thanksgiving ham. The best part is that no one will realize it's sugar free (unless you tell them). First, find a low-sugar ham locally. Most ham's are cured using some sugar, so do your best to find the lowest sugar option.

1 Half Spiral-Cut Ham

Maple Bourbon Glaze, prepared

If frozen, allow ham to completely thaw in refrigerator. This may take up to 72 hours.

Preheat oven to 350 °F.

Wrap a baking pan completely in foil.

Lay out additional foil on top of pan - enough to cover the ham.

Lay ham on foil flat side down and bring the foil up around the ham, covering it.

Make a small opening in the foil big enough to allow your meat thermometer to be inserted without making contact with the foil.

Insert the meat thermometer making sure not to insert it near the bone.

Place ham in oven. If your thermometer connects to your oven internally, make the connection at this time. If not, place the ham in a way that allows you to easily check the temperature by looking through the glass.

Bake at 350 °F until ham reaches 105F.

Remove ham from oven. Remove foil and baste with up to half of Bourbon Glaze.

Place ham (uncovered) back in oven and bake to 140 °F.

Remove ham from oven and baste with the remainder of the Bourbon Glaze.

Serve and enjoy.

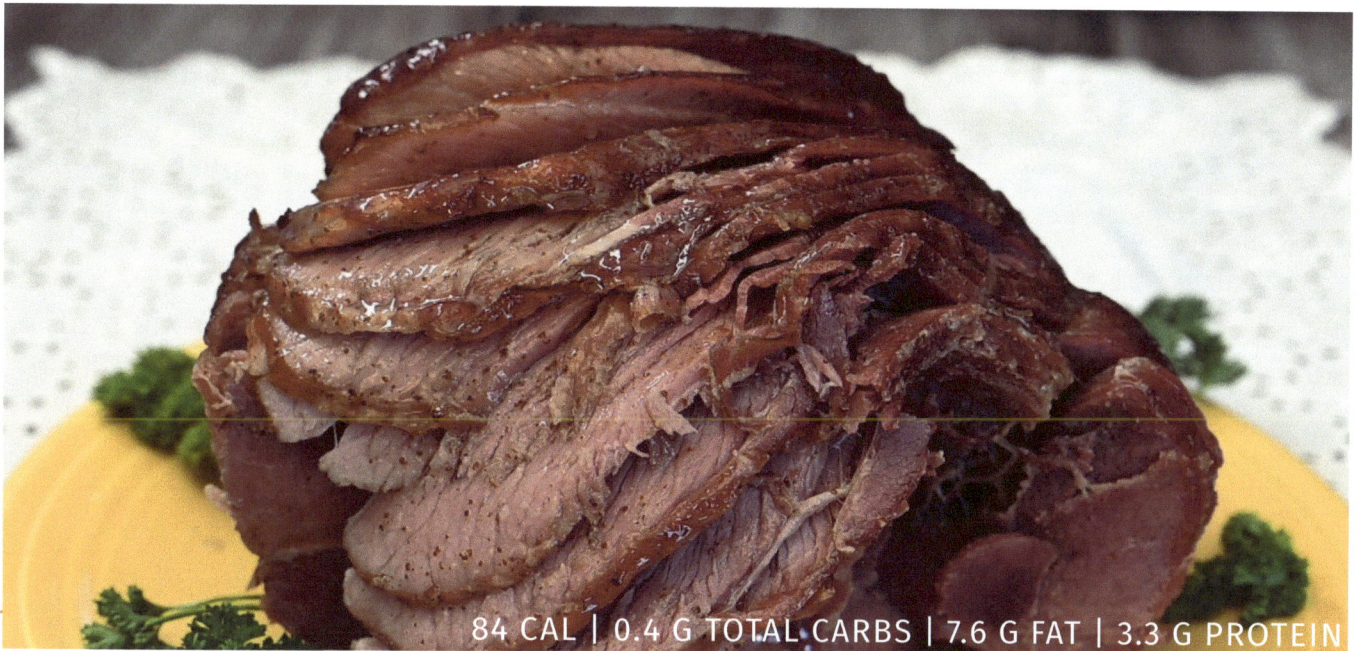

84 CAL | 0.4 G TOTAL CARBS | 7.6 G FAT | 3.3 G PROTEIN

YIELD: 1 CRUST

Easy Keto Press-In Pie Crust

This is my favorite keto pie crust because it takes just minutes to make and requires a lot less clean up than a traditional rolled-crust.

1 ½ cups (168 g) almond flour
5 Tablespoons butter, melted
1 Tablespoon sugar substitute
⅛ teaspoon xanthan gum

Recipe Tips: Xanthan gum is used as the binder in this crust. You can use guar gum as a replacement. You can use any sugar substitute here except for allulose. When using allulose, the pie crust tends to burn because allulose browns rapidly.

161 CALORIES | 3.7 G CARB
1.5 G FIBER | 2.1 G NET CARB
13.1 G FAT | 8.4 G PROTEIN

Grease the pie pan you wish to use with butter or coconut oil. Set aside.

In a medium-sized mixing bowl, stir together almond flour, xanthan gum, and sugar substitute until completely combined.

Drizzle in melted butter and stir until crumbly. The mixture should hold together when pressed.

Pour the crust mixture into your pie pan and spread around until evenly distributed across the pan with extra at the edges all the way around. Using your fingers or a plastic spoon, press the pie crust into the pan starting with the edges. Continue pressing until the pie crust covers the entire pan. If desired, shape the edges of the pie crust.

Now you're ready to fill or bake your crust. I highly recommend you use a pie shield when you bake this crust. Almond flour tends to brown very quickly and your edges may burn without a shield. You can fashion a pie shield yourself using aluminum foil or purchase some inexpensive shields to use over and over again.

To pre-bake the crust, place in a preheated 325 °F oven for 20-25 minutes until golden brown. Allow the crust to cool completely before filling.

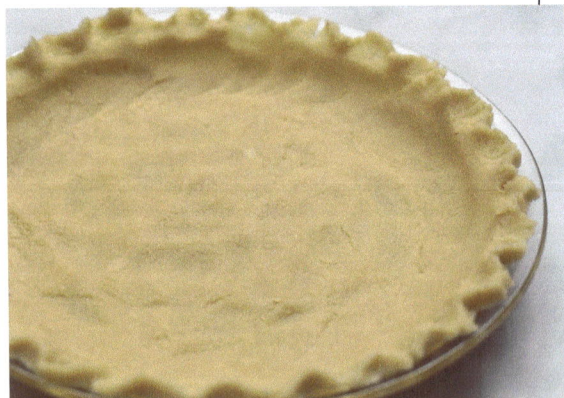

Hazelnut Pie Crust

For those that love a rolled-out pie crust, I've created this delicious crust using hazelnut flour, coconut flour, and tiger nut flour. You'll love this keto-friendly version of a traditional pie crust.

1 cup (112g) hazelnut flour
¼ cup (1 oz) coconut flour
½ cup (1 oz) tiger nut flour (or almond flour)
3 teaspoons granulated sugar substitute
½ cup cold butter (sliced)
1 large egg

Make the pie crust in your food processor or cut in the butter and then stir by hand.

In the bowl of your food processor, combine grain-free flours, granulated sugar substitute, and sliced cold butter. Use pulse to process the mixture until it resembles wet sand.

Add your egg to the mixture in the food processor and pulse together until combined.

Place your pie crust in a piece of parchment paper or plastic wrap, shaping it into a circular disc.

Refrigerate the pie crust for 30 minutes.

Preheat your oven to 350 °F if you are going to pre-bake the pie crust for a filled pie.

Remove the package from the fridge and roll out the pie crust between two sheets of parchment paper. If your crust warms a lot during the rolling, place it back in the fridge for a few minutes before attempting to put it on the pie pan. It will be challenging to handle if it's too warm.

Use the parchment paper to help you transfer the crust to a 9 inch pie plate. Patch as needed (the crust is very forgiving) and pinch your edges as you wish.

For a pre-baked pie crust: Bake in a 350 °F oven using pie crust shields (the edges will overbake without them) for 10-15 minutes or until lightly browned and cooked through.

188 CAL | 2.4 G NET CARB | 17.7 G FAT | 2.8 G PROTEIN

Keto Pecan Pie

Allulose is the super-star that makes this keto pecan pie recipe work. This is because allulose is a rare-sugar and cooks very similarly to real sugar. Know that allulose browns faster than real sugar which is why we remove the mixture from the heat right when the browning begins. To dress this pecan pie up more, sprinkle some sugar-free chocolate chips in the bottom of your pie crust before adding the filling.

¾ cup butter

1 cup allulose

½ cup sugar substitute

3 Tablespoons heavy
  whipping cream

½ teaspoon salt

1½ teaspoons xanthan gum

3 eggs

1 Tablespoon vanilla

2 cups chopped pecans

3 pecan halves for garnish

Prepare a 9-inch pie pan with the crust of your choice.

Preheat your oven to 350 °F.

Toast chopped pecans for 5 minutes in the oven, watching carefully so they don't burn.
Set aside.

In a large, heat-safe mixing bowl whisk egg until combined and lightened in color. Set aside.

In a medium-sized saucepan, melt butter over medium heat and then add allulose, sugar substitute, heavy cream, and salt. Cook over medium heat, stirring constantly, for 4-6 minutes until boiling and the mixture just begins to brown. Watch it very carefully and as soon as browning begins, immediately remove from the heat and continue stirring until bubbling goes away.

While whisking the egg mixture, pour a little bit of the hot mixture into the egg mixture.

Whisking constantly. This is called tempering. Pour the remaining hot liquid into the egg continuing to stir until completely combined.

While whisking the mixture, sprinkle in xanthan gum and add vanilla extract. Stir until the xanthan gum is completely combined. You may need to use an immersion blender or hand blender to get the xanthan gum to dissolve.

Finally, mix in the chopped pecans.

Pour mixture into prepared crust in your pie pan. Use three pecan halves to decorate the top.

Slide the pie pan onto a cookie sheet for easier transport into the oven.

Cover the edges of the pie crust with a baking shield or create a baking shield from foil.

Bake at 325 °F convection for 40 minutes. Allow the pie to cool completely before serving, about 2 hours.

Store in the refrigerator for up to 5 days.

30 CAL | 11.7 G CARB | 4.2 G FIBER | 1.3 G NET CARB | 3 G FAT | 1 G PROTEIN

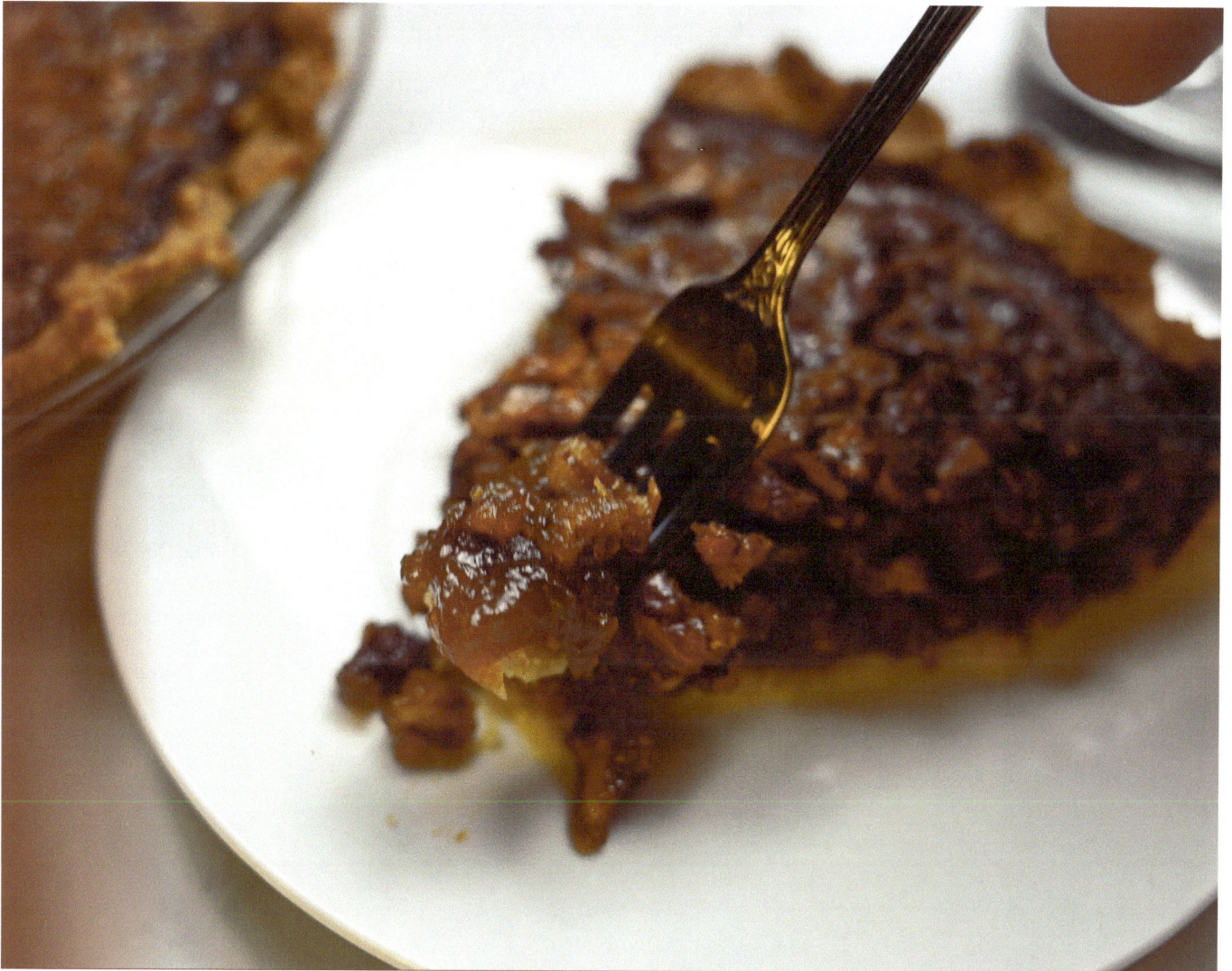

Low-carb Lemon Curd Pie

Our signature lemon pie features a tangy lemon curd filling topped with luxurious homemade whipped cream. This is sure to be a hit on your Thanksgiving table.

6 eggs, large
⅔ cup granulated sugar substitute
1 cup lemon juice (3-4 lemons)
12 Tablespoons unsalted butter
1 teaspoon vanilla extract
grated zest of two lemons

optional: 1 teaspoon lemon extract -or-
5-10 drops Young Living Lemon Vitality Essential Oil

Before you begin, prepare your tools so you can work quickly. Set the following items beside your stovetop.

- fine mesh colander to strain the lemon curd
- bowl to place under the colander to catch the curd

In a medium sized saucepan, with the heat off, mix eggs, granulated sugar substitute, and lemon zest together until thoroughly combined.

Mix in the lemon juice and butter and turn your heat to medium-low.

Whisk constantly over medium-low heat until mixture is thickened and comes to a gentle simmer. Allow the mixture to simmer only for a minute or two before removing from heat.

Working quickly, pour the lemon curd through the mesh colander. Use a spoon to work the curd through the colander.

Next, add your vanilla extract and optional lemon flavoring.

Taste-test the lemon curd and make any needed adjustments.

Allow the curd to cool for thirty minutes before pouring into your pre-baked pie shell. Place your pie in the refrigerator to chill thoroughly prior to topping with real whipped cream.

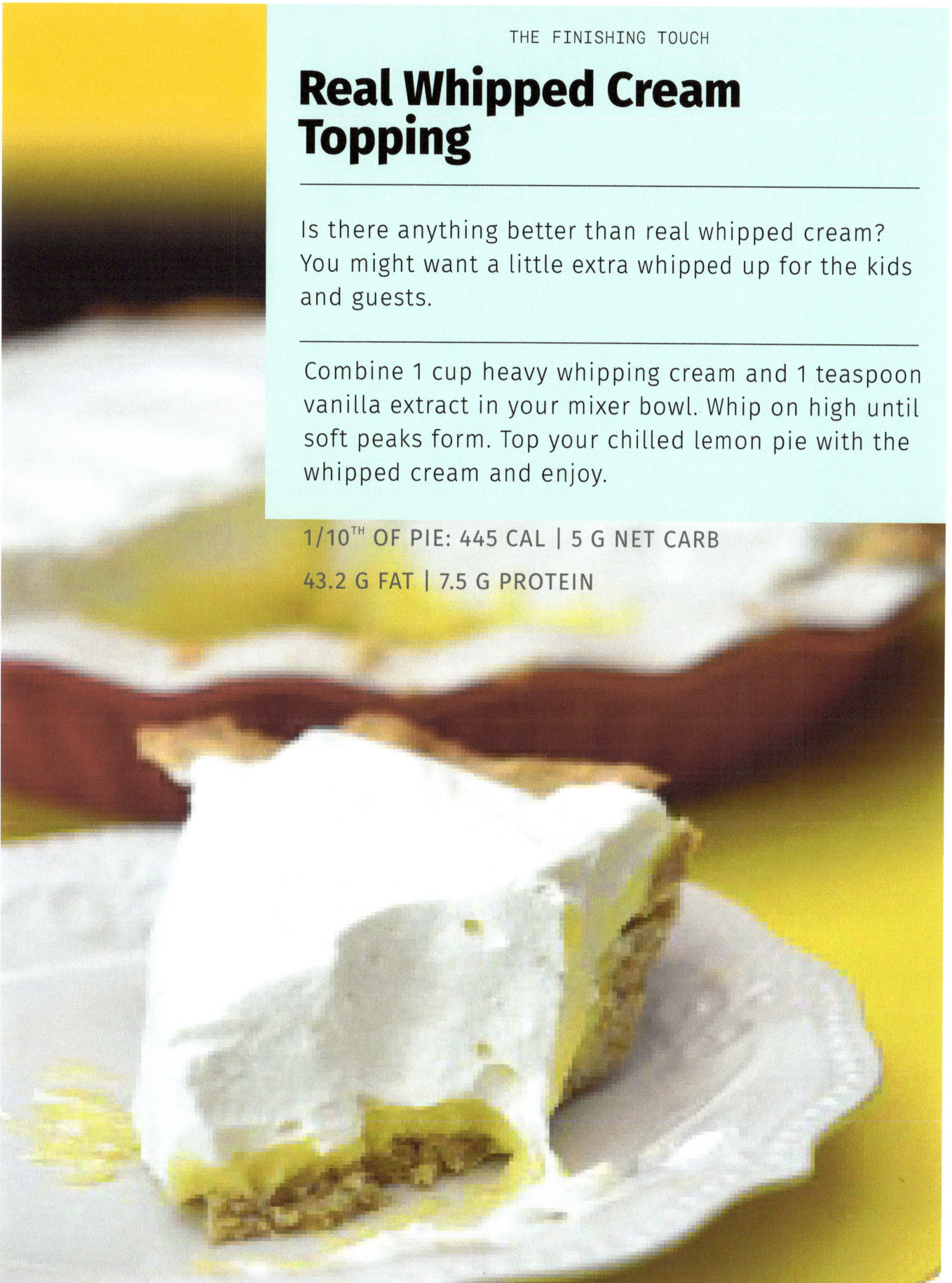

Real Whipped Cream Topping

Is there anything better than real whipped cream? You might want a little extra whipped up for the kids and guests.

Combine 1 cup heavy whipping cream and 1 teaspoon vanilla extract in your mixer bowl. Whip on high until soft peaks form. Top your chilled lemon pie with the whipped cream and enjoy.

1/10TH OF PIE: 445 CAL | 5 G NET CARB

43.2 G FAT | 7.5 G PROTEIN

Deep Dish Keto Pumpkin Pie

Our signature pumpkin pie is just as good as the full-sugar version. It pairs well with our press in almond flour crust or our hazelnut pie crust. We've used allulose and cooked it into the pumpkin to develop a deep brown sugar flavor we love in the best pumpkin pies. An alternate option is BochaSweet or stevia drops. Erythritol will want to crystalize in the pan and when leftovers are stored.

1 cup pumpkin purée

½ cup allulose

40 drops liquid stevia

1 teaspoon vanilla extract

1 Tablespoon ground cinnamon

1 teaspoon ground ginger

1 teaspoon ground nutmeg

¼ teaspoon ground cloves

½ teaspoon sea salt

⅔ cup heavy whipping cream

⅔ cup coconut cream

4 large eggs

Tip: Use a pie crust shield to prevent the edges of the crust from burning.

Prepare the pie crust and set aside.

Preheat oven to 325 °F.

In a medium-sized mixing bowl, combine heavy whipping cream and coconut cream. Set aside.

In a small saucepan, stir together pumpkin purée, allulose, stevia, vanilla, cinnamon, ginger, nutmeg, cloves, and salt.

Cook over medium heat for five minutes, stirring constantly. Allulose browns faster than sugar, so pay special attention that your pumpkin mixture doesn't burn.

Pour hot pumpkin mixture into the cream mixture and whisk until completely combined.

Whisk in eggs.

Pour pumpkin mixture into prepared pie shell.

Bake at 325 °F for 40 minutes or until the center is just slightly jiggly. Remove from oven and allow to cool completely. Store in the refrigerator for up to 3 days.

MACROS WITHOUT THE CRUST. DOES NOT INCLUDE SUGAR ALCOHOL.

159 CALORIES | 3.7 G CARBS | .8 G FIBER | 2.9 G NET CARB | 13.9 G FAT | 4 G PROTEIN

Spiced Whipped Cream

Top your dessert with this heavenly spiced whipped cream. When choosing cream at the store, choose a plain unadulterated heavy cream without added stabilizers. One cup of cream will whip into approximately 2 cups of whipped cream. To make this dairy free, use the same quantity of coconut cream. You will find coconut cream in the store on the shelf in a can or carton

1 cup heavy whipping cream
20 drops liquid stevia
⅛ teaspoon cinnamon
⅛ teaspoon nutmeg
1 teaspoon vanilla extract

Pour heavy whipping cream into a large, deep metal bowl that works with your mixer. Cover with plastic wrap and place in the freezer for 20-30 minutes.

Once chilled, remove from the freezer and add in the remaining ingredients.

Using your mixer's whisk attachment, whisk on medium speed until the first soft peaks appear. Turn mixer to low or finish by hand being careful not to over whisk the cream. Finished whipped cream should be soft and billowy. If the cream starts to become dense, you've over whipped it.

Cover and store in the refrigerator for up to 3 days. If the cream deflates in the fridge, simply whisk by hand until soft peaks re-form.

NUTRITION FACTS NOT INCLUDING SUGAR ALCOHOLS. PER 2 TABLESPOON SERVING.
51.4 CALORIES | .5 G CARB | 5.4 G FAT | .4 G PROTEIN

Pumpkin Bars with Cream Cheese Frosting

These grain-free pumpkin bars topped with cream cheese frosting are easy to make and have a texture that's reminiscent of pumpkin pie.

6 eggs

1 can (15 ounces) pumpkin puree

½ cup olive oil

1 cup sour cream

1 ½ Tablespoons pumpkin pie spice

1 Tablespoon pure vanilla extract

½ teaspoon almond extract

40 drops liquid stevia

1 teaspoon molasses

⅓ cup (54g) coconut flour

¼ teaspoon xanthan gum

1 teaspoon baking soda

¼ teaspoon cream of tarter

Preheat oven to 350 °F.

In a large mixing bowl, whisk together eggs, pumpkin, olive oil, sour cream, pumpkin pie spice, vanilla extract, almond extract, sugar substitute, stevia, and molasses until thoroughly combined.

Next, whisk or beat in the coconut flour and xanthan gum. Allow mixture to rest for 3-5 minutes while you prepare a 9x9 baking pan by greasing it heavily with coconut oil or butter. You'll notice the batter has thickened considerably as the coconut flour absorbs moisture.

Mix in the baking soda and cream of tartar and then pour batter into prepared 9x9 baking dish. Bake at 350 °F for 30 minutes until a toothpick inserted into the center comes out clean.

Cool completely and top with cream cheese frosting.

To make the cream cheese frosting, combine ¼ cup softened butter, 8 ounces softened cream cheese, ½ cup warmed heavy whipping cream, ¼ cup sugar substitute, 30 drops stevia, 2 teaspoon vanilla and 1 teaspoon maple extract in a large mixing bowl. Using your blender, mix on low speed until ingredients are combined. Then whip on high speed until light and fluffy. **Note: You must warm your ingredients for them to whip correctly.**

247 CALORIES | 4.4 G NET CARB | 22.5 G FAT | 4.6 G PROTEIN

Discover Our Other Cookbooks & Resources

- ☑ Keto Planners
- ☑ Keto Tear-Off Pads
- ☑ Inspirational Journals

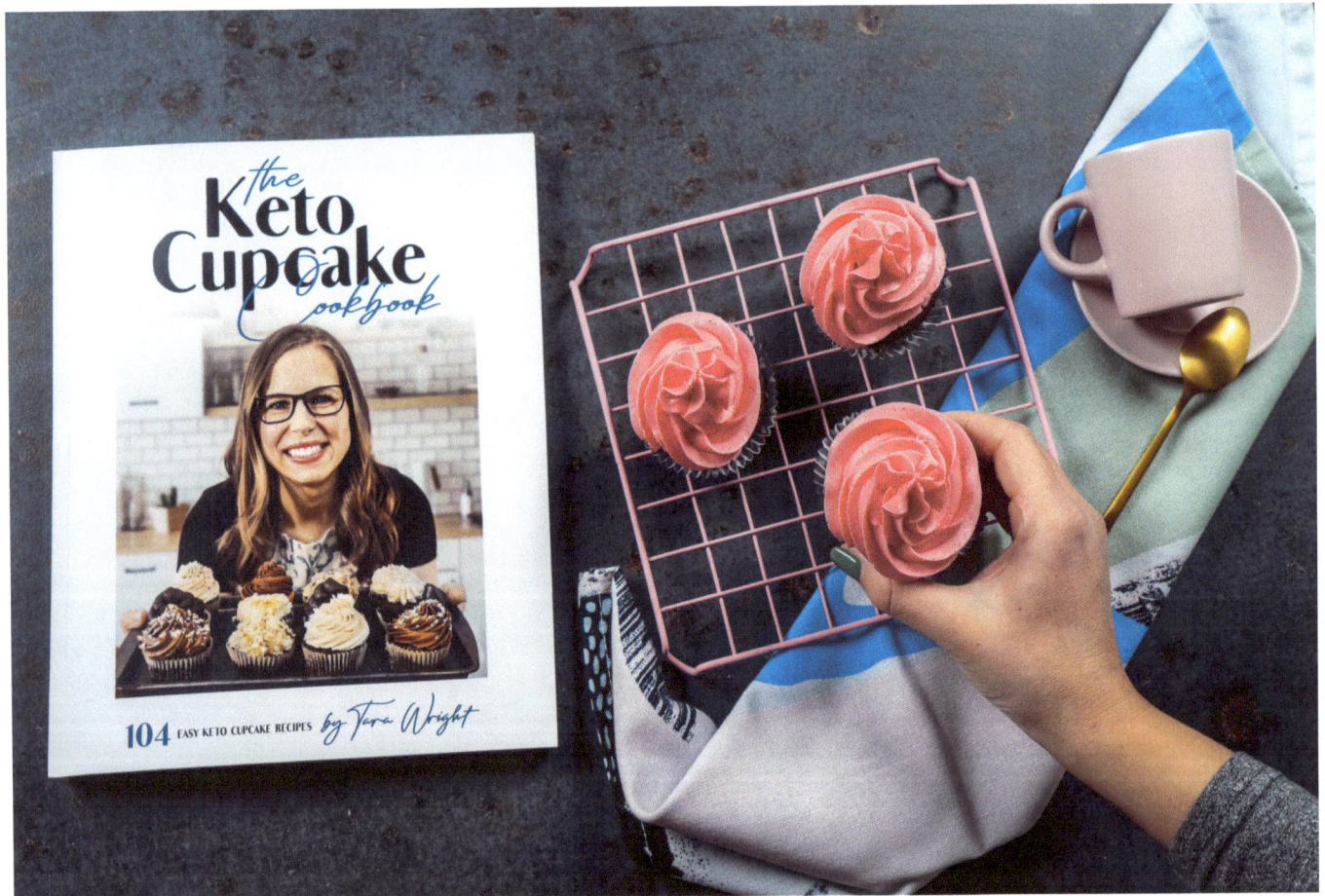

SAVE 10% WITH COUPON CODE

THANKS10

www.sustainableketo.com

www.ingramcontent.com/pod-product-compliance
Lightning Source LLC
Chambersburg PA
CBHW040021050426
42452CB00002B/84